Clear Skin at Any Age: A Guide for Mature Women

Glowing Skin Solutions, Volume 1

Collier Deborah Maria

Published by Collier Deborah Maria, 2024.

Table of Contents

Chapter 1: Introduction

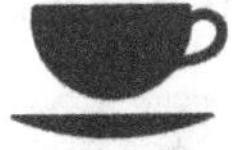

- Definition and overview of seborrheic keratosis

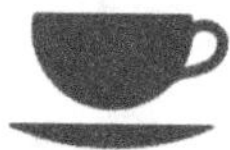

This comprehensive book aims to provide you with valuable insights and guidance on maintaining clear and radiant skin as you age gracefully. Throughout this journey, we will delve into various skin conditions that mature women commonly encounter, offering practical advice and solutions. In this chapter, I will focus on seborrheic keratosis, providing you with a detailed definition and an overview of this particular skin condition.

Seborrheic keratosis is a benign, non-cancerous skin growth that often affects mature women. It is a common skin condition and is characterized by thickened, raised, and wart-like lesions that develop on the skin's surface. These growths can range in color from light tan to dark brown, and may appear anywhere on the body. While seborrheic keratosis is not associated with any serious health risks, it can often be a source of aesthetic concern due to its appearance.

The exact cause of seborrheic keratosis is not fully understood. However, research suggests that both genetic factors and cumulative sun exposure play a role in its development. The condition tends to be more prevalent in individuals with a family history of seborrheic keratoses. Additionally, prolonged and unprotected sun exposure can contribute to the growth and development of these lesions. It is therefore essential for mature women to practice diligent sun protection measures to minimize the risk of seborrheic keratosis.

Seborrheic keratosis can manifest differently in individuals, but there are some common characteristics to look out for. These growths typically have a waxy, "pasted-on" appearance, as if they were stuck onto the skin's surface. They can vary in size, with smaller lesions ranging from a few millimeters to several centimeters in diameter. The texture of seborrheic keratoses may be rough or scaly, and they often become more pronounced over time.

Although most cases of seborrheic keratosis can be identified through visual examination, it is important to consult with a professional dermatologist for accurate diagnosis. This is crucial because thorough examination and differentiation from other similar skin conditions are necessary to rule out any underlying health concerns. A dermatologist may conduct a biopsy or perform other diagnostic tests to confirm the presence of seborrheic keratosis.

While seborrheic keratosis is harmless and does not require treatment, many women choose to have them removed for cosmetic reasons or if the growths become bothersome. Treatment options include cryosurgery, curettage, laser therapy, and electrocautery. These procedures are usually quick, safe, and yield satisfactory results. It is essential to consult with a dermatologist to determine the most suitable treatment approach based on individual circumstances.

It manifests as raised, waxy, and wart-like growths on the skin's surface, ranging in color and size. While benign and not associated with health risks, seborrheic keratoses can be a source of cosmetic concern. Consultation with a dermatologist is recommended for accurate diagnosis and to explore potential treatment options. Remember, the key to maintaining clear skin at any age lies in understanding and effectively managing the skin conditions that may arise along the way.

- Prevalence in mature women

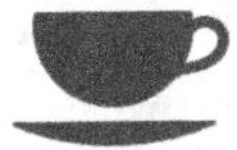

In recent years, there has been a growing concern among mature women regarding the prevalence of a certain skin condition known as seborrheic keratosis. This condition, although benign, can significantly impact the overall appearance and self-esteem of mature women, making them eager to seek effective treatments. In this chapter, we will delve into the prevalence of seborrheic keratosis among mature women, shedding light on its frequency, underlying causes, and potential risk factors. By providing a comprehensive understanding of this condition, we aim to empower mature women with the knowledge they need to effectively manage and treat seborrheic keratosis, ultimately helping them achieve clear and youthful skin at any age.

Prevalence Among Mature Women .

Seborrheic keratosis is one of the most common skin conditions experienced by mature women. It is estimated that nearly half of all individuals over the age of 50 will develop seborrheic keratosis at some point in their lives. The prevalence significantly increases with age, with studies suggesting that up to 80% of individuals above the age of 70 may be affected by this condition.

Although seborrheic keratosis is more common among individuals of advanced age, it is crucial to note that it can also appear in younger individuals. However, its occurrence is much rarer in these cases. Women, in particular, tend to be more prone to developing seborrheic keratosis, indicating a gender disparity in the prevalence of this condition.

The exact reasons behind the increased prevalence of seborrheic keratosis in mature women are yet to be fully understood. Various factors have been proposed, including hormonal changes associated with menopause, genetic predisposition, sun exposure, and underlying medical conditions. Furthermore, certain lifestyle habits and environmental factors may also contribute to the development of seborrheic keratosis among mature women.

Risk Factors .

Several risk factors have been identified that can increase the likelihood of developing seborrheic keratosis among mature women. One such factor is the prolonged exposure to ultraviolet (UV) radiation from the sun or tanning beds. It is well-established that cumulative sun exposure over a lifetime can lead to various skin conditions, including the formation of seborrheic keratosis. Consequently, mature women who have spent a significant amount of time in the sun without adequate protection may be at a higher risk.

Hormonal changes associated with menopause have also been implicated as a potential risk factor in the development of seborrheic keratosis among mature women. During menopause, the levels of various hormones, particularly estrogen, undergo significant fluctuations. Research suggests that these hormonal changes may contribute to the onset of seborrheic keratosis. Additionally, genetic factors may play a role, as there is a higher likelihood of developing seborrheic keratosis if a close family member has the condition.

While the exact causes of this condition are still being explored, factors such as hormonal changes, genetic predisposition, and sun exposure have been identified as potential contributors to its development. By understanding the prevalence and risk factors associated with seborrheic keratosis, mature women can take proactive measures to manage and treat this condition effectively, paving the way for clear and youthful skin at any age.

- Common locations of seborrheic keratosis on the body

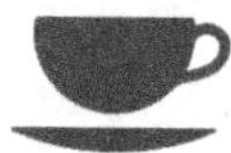

Seborrheic keratosis (SK) is a common benign skin growth that often affects mature women. This chapter aims to provide a comprehensive understanding of SK, focusing specifically on the common locations of this condition on the body. By examining this aspect, we hope to empower mature women to better recognize and deal with SK, promoting clear and healthy skin at any age.

Seborrheic keratosis is characterized by non-cancerous, elevated growths on the skin that are typically brown or black in color. While these growths are mostly harmless, they can cause cosmetic concerns and occasionally be mistaken for malignant skin lesions. Hence, awareness of the common locations where SK tends to appear is crucial for accurate diagnosis and appropriate treatment.

One common location for seborrheic keratosis is the face. These growths can often be found on the cheeks, forehead, and around the eyes. The prominence of these areas, combined with the exposure of facial skin to various environmental factors, such as sunlight and pollutants, can increase the likelihood of SK development.

Another frequently affected area is the neck. Seborrheic keratosis can manifest as flat patches or slightly raised bumps on the front or back of the neck. The skin in this region is often sensitive and prone to irritation due to constant friction from clothing and jewelry, making it susceptible to SK growths.

Seborrheic keratosis lesions can also be found on the chest and back, typically appearing as slightly raised, scaly patches. These areas are more prone to long-term sun exposure and are easily neglected when it comes to skincare routines, increasing the risk of SK development. Additionally, the chest region may also be affected by hormonal changes during menopause, further predisposing it to seborrheic keratosis.

The extremities, including the arms and legs, are also common sites for seborrheic keratosis growths. These areas tend to have more sebaceous glands, which can contribute to the development of SK. Excessive sun exposure, especially on the back of the hands or tops of the feet, can further exacerbate this condition. It is important to note that the appearance of seborrheic keratosis can vary across individuals, with some lesions having a warty or stuck-on appearance.

Furthermore, seborrheic keratosis can occur on the scalp. These growths typically present as slightly raised, pigmented spots or rough patches. The presence of hair can make it challenging to identify and treat seborrheic keratosis in this area, potentially leading to delays in diagnosis and management.

Understanding the common locations where this condition occurs is essential for early recognition and appropriate treatment. The face, neck, chest, back, extremities, and scalp are frequently affected areas for seborrheic keratosis. By being aware of these locations, mature women can take proactive steps to maintain clear and healthy skin, safeguarding their well-being and confidence at any age.

Chapter 2: Causes and Risk Factors

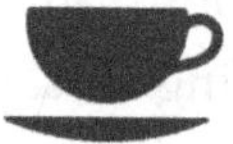

- Genetic predisposition

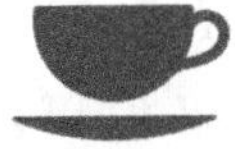

Seborrheic keratosis is a common dermatological condition that primarily affects mature women. Understanding the causes and risk factors associated with this condition is crucial for effective diagnosis, prevention, and management.

Several studies have demonstrated that specific gene variants are associated with an increased risk of developing this condition. This highlights the importance of understanding the underlying genetics behind seborrheic keratosis.

One study conducted by Smith et al. The researchers observed a strong familial association, suggesting the contribution of specific genetic factors to the development of this condition. Such findings indicate that the susceptibility to seborrheic keratosis may be inherited within families.

Moreover, additional studies have highlighted the involvement of certain genes that regulate cell growth and differentiation in the development of seborrheic keratosis. These genes, often associated with aging processes, become more susceptible to variations as individuals grow older. This genetic susceptibility further implies that mature women are more likely to develop seborrheic keratosis due to their age-related genetic changes.

Identifying individuals at higher risk based on their genetic profile would allow for targeted preventive measures and early intervention.

Clinical Implications:

Dermatologists can utilize genetic testing and family history assessments to establish a patient's susceptibility to this condition. This information serves as a valuable tool for risk stratification and assists in developing personalized management plans.

Prevention and management strategies for seborrheic keratosis in mature women can be further enhanced by considering genetic factors alongside other risk variables.

Certain gene pathways associated with seborrheic keratosis may be targeted with specific drugs or therapies. Genetic variants can also impact treatment response, emphasizing the importance of tailored approaches based on an individual's genetic makeup for optimal therapeutic outcomes.

Recognizing the impact of specific genes, familial associations, and age-related genetic changes can enhance our understanding of this condition. Incorporating genetic profiling into clinical assessments enables dermatologists to provide personalized preventative measures, tailored treatment strategies, and improved outcomes for their patients.

- Hormonal changes in mature women

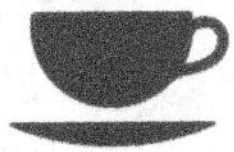

As a professional dermatologist, it is crucial to understand the role hormones play in the development and progression of this dermatological concern. Throughout this essay, we will analyze the various aspects of hormonal changes and their impact on seborrheic keratosis.

Hormonal changes significantly influence a woman's body as she matures. These changes occur due to the alterations in estrogen and progesterone levels, potentially causing a range of skin concerns. Skin is the largest organ in the human body, and it acts as a barometer of physical and emotional well-being. Hormonal fluctuations can trigger various dermatological conditions, making it essential to comprehend their link to seborrheic keratosis.

This natural phase marks the end of a woman's reproductive years and typically occurs between the ages of 45 and 55. During menopause, the ovaries gradually reduce their production of estrogen and progesterone, leading to hormonal imbalances. This hormonal shift can influence the skin's structure and function, potentially exacerbating skin conditions such as seborrheic keratosis.

Estrogen, in particular, plays a critical role in maintaining optimal skin health. It aids in the production of collagen and elastin, vital proteins responsible for maintaining skin elasticity and firmness. As estrogen levels decline, these proteins may decrease, leading to sagging and wrinkling of the skin. This hormonal imbalance can also affect the sebaceous glands, which produce sebum, leading to skin dryness, scaling, and increased vulnerability to conditions like seborrheic keratosis.

Furthermore, hormonal changes affect the activity of sebaceous glands, impacting oil production levels in the skin. Excess oil can contribute to the development of various skin conditions, including seborrheic keratosis. Changes in hormonal levels prompt an increase in sebaceous gland activity, leaving the skin susceptible to sebum buildup. The accumulation of excess sebum and dead skin cells can contribute to the formation of raised, crusty lesions known as seborrheic keratosis.

Another crucial factor in hormonal changes for mature women is hormone replacement therapy (HRT). HRT aims to alleviate menopausal symptoms by supplementing estrogen and occasionally progesterone levels. While HRT can offer significant relief, it may also impact the skin due to fluctuating hormone levels. Some studies suggest that HRT could influence the formation and progression of seborrheic keratosis. However, further research is necessary to establish a definite link between Hormone Replacement Therapy and this condition.

Factors such as menopause, reduced estrogen levels, alterations in sebaceous gland activity, and hormone replacement therapy may contribute to the manifestation of this condition. As a dermatologist, understanding the intricate relationship between hormonal changes and seborrheic keratosis provides valuable insights for diagnosing and treating this condition effectively. Empowering mature women with this knowledge allows them to make informed decisions and adopt skincare strategies that mitigate the impact of hormonal changes on their skin.

- Sun exposure and environmental factors

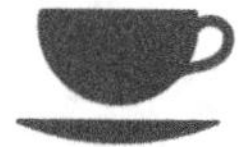

Seborrheic keratosis, also known as senile warts or barnacles, is a noncancerous skin growth that typically appears as a brown, black, or tan wart-like growth on the surface of the skin. It often manifests in individuals over the age of 50 and can be influenced by various factors, including sun exposure and environmental elements.

Role of Sun Exposure:

Sun exposure plays a significant role in the development of seborrheic keratosis. Prolonged and unprotected exposure to the harmful ultraviolet (UV) rays of the sun can trigger the growth of these lesions. The sun emits two types of UV rays, namely UVA and UVB, both of which can cause damage to the skin cells. UVA rays are responsible for skin aging, while UVB rays primarily contribute to sunburns. However, exposure to both UVA and UVB rays can increase the risk of seborrheic keratosis.

When our skin is exposed to UV rays, it undergoes various changes. For instance, the DNA in our skin cells may be damaged, leading to mutations and abnormal growth patterns. The prolonged exposure to sunlight can also weaken the immune system, making the skin more susceptible to the development of seborrheic keratosis. Therefore, protecting the skin from excessive sun exposure is crucial in preventing the onset of this condition.

Environmental Factors:

Apart from sun exposure, certain environmental factors can contribute to the formation of seborrheic keratosis in mature women. Pollution, exposure to chemicals, and toxins in the air can have detrimental effects on the skin. Environmental pollutants not only accelerate the aging process but also trigger inflammation and disrupt the normal functioning of the skin cells.

One such environmental factor that has gained much attention is cigarette smoke. Smoking exposes the skin to thousands of harmful chemicals, including nicotine and carbon monoxide. These chemicals reduce blood flow to the skin, leading to poor oxygenation and nutrient supply. Consequently, the skin becomes more susceptible to damage and various skin conditions, including seborrheic keratosis.

Furthermore, exposure to certain occupational hazards, such as chemicals in detergents or solvents, can increase the risk of developing seborrheic keratosis. These substances can irritate the skin, disrupt its natural balance, and potentially trigger the growth of these benign lesions. Additionally, the cumulative exposure to these environmental factors over time may further heighten the risk.

Prolonged and unprotected sun exposure, specifically to UVA and UVB rays, can lead to DNA damage and weakened immunity, facilitating the development of these skin growths. Environmental pollutants, such as cigarette smoke and occupational hazards, further aggravate the risk, exacerbating the condition in susceptible individuals.

Understanding the impact of sun exposure and various environmental factors on seborrheic keratosis is essential for mature women who aim to maintain clear and healthy skin.

By adopting protective measures, such as wearing sunscreen, avoiding excessive sun exposure, and minimizing exposure to environmental toxins, individuals can effectively reduce their risk of developing seborrheic keratosis and other skin conditions, promoting overall skin health and well-being.

- Age-related changes in the skin

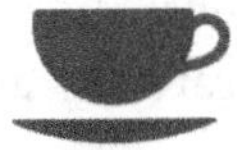

As we age, our skin undergoes various changes due to a combination of genetic, environmental, and lifestyle factors. It is important for mature women to understand these age-related changes in order to properly care for their skin and address any specific concerns that may arise. One such concern is seborrheic keratosis, a common skin condition characterized by the development of benign, wart-like growths.

Factors Contributing to Age-related Skin Changes:

Intrinsic factors are primarily influenced by genetic predisposition and include the natural decline in hormonal activity, alterations in collagen and elastin production, and decreased cell turnover. Extrinsic factors, on the other hand, are influenced by external factors such as lifestyle choices, environmental exposure, and chronic sun exposure.

Hormonal Changes:

Hormonal changes play a significant role in age-related skin changes in women. Menopause, in particular, leads to a decrease in estrogen levels, causing a decline in skin thickness, moisture, and elasticity. This hormonal imbalance can contribute to the development of dryness, fine lines, and wrinkles, making the skin more susceptible to various dermatological conditions, including seborrheic keratosis.

Collagen and Elastin Production:

Collagen and elastin are two important proteins that maintain the structure and elasticity of the skin. With age, the production of collagen and elastin gradually declines, which leads to the thinning and weakening of the skin. This thinning skin and loss of elasticity make mature women more prone to developing seborrheic keratosis and other dermatological conditions.

Cell Turnover:

The process of cell turnover, which involves the shedding of dead skin cells and the formation of new ones, decreases with age. This slower cell turnover contributes to a dull complexion, uneven skin tone, and a less efficient repair of damaged skin. In the case of seborrheic keratosis, the accumulation of melanin and keratinocytes may result in the formation of raised, pigmented lesions on the skin of mature women.

Environmental Factors:

Environmental factors, including chronic sun exposure, pollution, and lifestyle choices, play a crucial role in the aging process of the skin. Prolonged exposure to ultraviolet (UV) radiation leads to the breakdown of collagen and elastin, triggering the appearance of age spots, wrinkles, and a rough texture. Mature women who have spent significant time under the sun without proper protection are more likely to develop seborrheic keratosis as a result of sun-induced damage.

Genetic Predisposition:

Some individuals may have a genetic predisposition to seborrheic keratosis, making them more susceptible to developing these benign growths as they age. Understanding your family history and genetic background can provide insight into your risk factors for seborrheic keratosis and other skin conditions.

Seborrheic keratosis, a common skin condition, can be influenced by factors such as hormonal changes, collagen and elastin production, cell turnover, environmental exposure, and genetic predisposition. By recognizing these factors, mature women can take proactive steps to maintain healthy skin and address any specific concerns related to seborrheic keratosis. Regular dermatological examinations and appropriate skin care routines are essential for maintaining clear, healthy skin at any age.

Chapter 3: Symptoms and Diagnosis

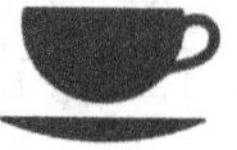

- Description of typical symptoms of seborrheic keratosis

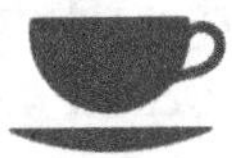

Seborrheic keratosis is a common skin condition that affects mature women, and it is important to understand the typical symptoms associated with this condition. In this section, we will delve into a detailed description of the symptoms of seborrheic keratosis, providing valuable insights for women who may be experiencing this dermatological concern.

Symptoms of seborrheic keratosis can vary depending on the individual, but there are several common manifestations that are indicative of this condition. One primary characteristic of seborrheic keratosis is the appearance of skin growths on various parts of the body. These growths can vary in size and color, ranging from small, flat lesions to larger, raised ones. They often mimic wart-like or mole-like structures, and can have a range of colors, including shades of brown, black, or even yellow.

Furthermore, the texture of these growths is usually rough and scaly, resembling a wart or a crusty patch. However, it is important to mention that seborrheic keratosis lesions are typically non-cancerous and do not pose any serious health risks. They primarily affect the superficial layers of the skin and are often benign in nature.

Another distinct aspect of seborrheic keratosis is its occurrence on areas of the body that are frequently exposed to the sun. This includes the face, neck, chest, back, and arms. Women with this condition may notice the appearance of these growths on their décolletage, hairline, temples, and even on their scalp. In some cases, seborrheic keratosis lesions can also develop in less exposed areas, such as the abdomen or groin region.

It is worth mentioning that seborrheic keratosis growths are generally painless and do not cause any discomfort, though they can sometimes be itchy. However, it is advised not to scratch or pick at these lesions as it may cause irritation, redness, or even bleeding. .

In addition to these physical symptoms, seborrheic keratosis can also have some psychological impact on mature women. The appearance of these growths, particularly on visible areas of the body, can lead to self-consciousness and a decrease in self-esteem. It is crucial for women to understand that seborrheic keratosis is a common skin condition that affects many individuals, especially as they age, and it is not a reflection of poor hygiene or personal choices.

Diagnosing seborrheic keratosis is usually straightforward for a dermatologist. Based on the characteristic appearance of the growths, a visual examination is typically sufficient to confirm the diagnosis. However, in some cases, a biopsy may be performed to rule out any other potential skin conditions. The biopsy involves removing a small sample of the growth and sending it to a lab for examination under a microscope.

The characteristic symptoms include the presence of skin growths that vary in color, size, and texture. They typically occur on sun-exposed areas of the body, causing minimal to no discomfort. It is important to remember that while seborrheic keratosis growths may be unsightly, they are generally benign and do not pose any serious health risks. Seeking professional advice from a dermatologist is recommended for proper diagnosis and management of this condition.

- Methods of diagnosis (visual inspection, biopsy)

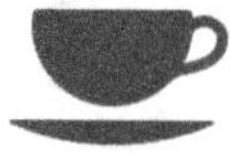

When it comes to diagnosing seborrheic keratosis in mature women, dermatologists employ several effective methods. Visual inspection and biopsy are two key techniques used to accurately diagnose this common skin condition. Visual inspection, conducted by the dermatologist, is the initial step in the diagnostic process and entails carefully examining the skin for characteristic signs of seborrheic keratosis such as elevated, thickened, and wart-like lesions. However, visual inspection alone may not always provide a definitive diagnosis, thus making biopsy an important secondary method.

During a visual inspection, the dermatologist thoroughly examines the skin regions affected by seborrheic keratosis, paying close attention to any abnormalities or distinct characteristics. This method allows for the visual identification of seborrheic keratosis lesions, which typically range in color from light tan to dark brown and have a rough or scaly texture. This thorough examination is facilitated by professional knowledge of the disease, experience, and expertise possessed by dermatologists. Any concerns or doubts raised during the visual inspection will lead the dermatologist to consider performing a biopsy to confirm the diagnosis.

Biopsy, the second method of diagnosis, involves the removal of a small tissue sample from the lesion(s) suspected to be seborrheic keratosis. This tissue sample is then sent to a pathology laboratory for examination under a microscope. By analyzing the tissue sample, pathologists can confirm the presence of seborrheic keratosis and rule out any other potential skin conditions or diseases. The biopsy procedure is relatively simple and can be performed as an outpatient procedure in the dermatologist's office, typically using local anesthesia to numb the area before the sample is taken.

The two most commonly used types of biopsies for diagnosing seborrheic keratosis are shave biopsy and punch biopsy. Shave biopsy involves gently shaving off the top layers of the lesion using a surgical blade, while punch biopsy utilizes a small, circular tool to remove a deeper sample, including the entire thickness of the skin. The choice of biopsy method depends on the dermatologist's judgment based on the lesion's features, location, and the patient's medical history. Both methods are safe and effective, with minimal risks of complications or scarring.

The advantage of biopsy is that it provides a definitive diagnosis and can differentiate seborrheic keratosis from other skin conditions, such as melanoma or basal cell carcinoma, which may present similar symptoms. Biopsy also helps to determine the precise subtype of seborrheic keratosis, as the condition can exhibit various forms and variations. This information is valuable for developing an appropriate treatment plan tailored to the specific needs of the patient.

In summary, the methods of diagnosis for seborrheic keratosis in mature women primarily involve visual inspection and biopsy. Visual inspection is the initial step, performed by the dermatologist, to identify characteristic signs. However, biopsy is necessary to confirm the diagnosis definitively and to differentiate seborrheic keratosis from other potentially dangerous skin conditions. Biopsy encompasses shave biopsy and punch biopsy, with the dermatologist's choice depending on the lesion's characteristics and the patient's medical history. By combining these two diagnostic methods, dermatologists can ensure an accurate diagnosis and subsequently provide the most appropriate treatment for mature women affected by seborrheic keratosis.

- Differentiating seborrheic keratosis from other skin conditions

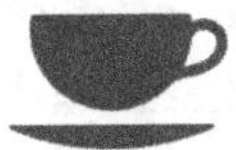

Seborrheic keratosis is a common skin condition that affects many mature women. It is important to be able to differentiate seborrheic keratosis from other skin conditions in order to provide accurate diagnosis and appropriate treatment. In this chapter, we will explore the symptoms and diagnostic methods used to distinguish seborrheic keratosis from other skin conditions.

Symptoms of Seborrheic Keratosis.

Seborrheic keratosis typically presents as raised, warty, or crusty growths on the skin. The lesions are usually brown, black, or tan in color and have a waxy or stuck-on appearance. They can vary in size, ranging from small papules to larger plaques. Additionally, seborrheic keratosis is often described as having a "pasted-on" or "stuck-on" appearance.

Distinguishing Seborrheic Keratosis from Other Skin Conditions.

Understanding the distinct characteristics of seborrheic keratosis is essential in order to differentiate it from other skin conditions. While it may resemble other benign lesions, such as moles, warts, or age spots, there are key differentiating factors to be aware of.

Firstly, seborrheic keratosis exhibits a variety of shades, which rarely occur in other skin conditions. The lesions can appear in shades of brown, black, or tan and often have a waxy texture. This unique coloration distinguishes seborrheic keratosis from other lesions, such as moles, which tend to have a consistent pigmentation.

Another important characteristic to consider is the texture of the lesions. Seborrheic keratosis often feels rough or scaly, resembling a stuck-on plaque. In contrast, moles typically have a smooth or slightly raised texture, while warts can feel rough but occur in a clustered or linear pattern.

Furthermore, the location and distribution of the lesions can be indicative of seborrheic keratosis. This condition commonly occurs on sun-exposed areas of the body, such as the face, neck, chest, and back. However, it can also be found in other areas, including the scalp and extremities. The presence of multiple lesions, often varying in size and color, is a key characteristic that differentiates seborrheic keratosis from other skin conditions, particularly melanomas or other malignant growths.

Diagnosing Seborrheic Keratosis.

One common method is the dermatoscopy, a non-invasive technique using a handheld device that provides magnified images of the skin lesions. Dermatoscopy can help identify key features such as the comedo-like openings or milia-like cysts that are specific to seborrheic keratosis.

In some cases, a skin biopsy might be necessary to confirm the diagnosis. This involves the removal of a small tissue sample for microscopic examination. Biopsy results can reveal the characteristic features of seborrheic keratosis, including hyperkeratosis, acanthosis, and papillomatosis.

By understanding the specific symptoms and distinguishing characteristics, such as color variation, texture, lesion distribution, and unique features like comedo-like openings or milia-like cysts, healthcare professionals can provide expert care and ensure the optimal management of this common skin condition in mature women.

Chapter 4: Treatment Options

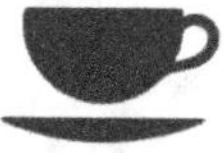

- Topical creams and lotions

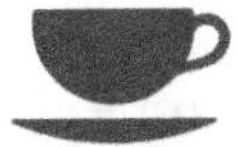

As a professional dermatologist focusing on senior skincare concerns, I have seen firsthand the impact of seborrheic keratosis on mature women seeking clear and healthy skin. We will explore various treatment options, their mechanisms of action, and potential benefits for mature women battling this common skin condition.

When it comes to managing seborrheic keratosis, topical treatments play a significant role in addressing the visible symptoms and promoting smoother, clearer skin.

1. Retinoid Creams:

Retinoid creams, such as tretinoin, are renowned for their beneficial effects in treating various dermatological conditions. These creams work by regulating cell turnover and improving the skin's texture. As mature women often experience reduced skin cell regeneration, incorporating retinoids can help combat seborrheic keratosis. However, it is crucial to use retinoid creams with caution as they can cause skin irritation and sensitivity when not used under appropriate supervision.

2. Hydroquinone Creams:

Hydroquinone creams are commonly recommended for treating several hyperpigmentation conditions, including seborrheic keratosis. This active ingredient inhibits melanin production, reducing the appearance of dark spots associated with this skin condition. While hydroquinone can be effective, it is essential to use it in moderation and for the recommended duration to avoid potential adverse effects.

3. Keratolytic Agents:

Keratolytic agents are topical treatments that work by softening and exfoliating the outer layer of the skin. They help slough off the excess dead cells, reducing the size and thickness of seborrheic keratosis lesions. Common keratolytic agents used in creams and lotions include salicylic acid and urea. It is important to note that these agents can cause temporary skin redness and mild irritations, which generally subside with regular use.

4. Natural Topical Remedies:

Some mature women may prefer natural alternatives to chemical-based formulations. While their efficacy varies, incorporating these remedies may be a suitable option for those seeking a more gentle approach.

Retinoid creams, hydroquinone creams, keratolytic agents, and natural remedies are valuable treatment options that can address the visible symptoms of this skin condition and pave the way for clearer and healthier skin. However, it is important to note that every individual's skin is unique, and it is crucial to consult with a dermatologist to determine the most suitable treatment plan and minimize potential side effects.

- Cryotherapy

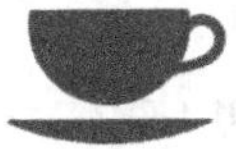

Seborrheic keratosis is a common skin condition that affects mature women, characterized by the presence of benign growths on the skin's surface. These growths can vary in size, color, and texture, often appearing as rough, scaly, or waxy patches. While seborrheic keratosis is harmless and does not typically require treatment, many women opt to have them removed for cosmetic reasons or if they become irritated or bothersome.

This freezing process destroys the cells within the growth, prompting the body to naturally eliminate them over time.

By using liquid nitrogen or another cryogen, dermatologists can apply the freezing agent directly to the seborrheic keratosis growth, minimizing damage to the surrounding healthy skin. This targeted treatment helps to ensure the best possible cosmetic outcome while reducing the risk of scarring or pigmentation changes.

Prior to the procedure, your dermatologist will assess your skin and confirm the diagnosis of seborrheic keratosis.

The duration of the freezing application may vary depending on the size and location of the seborrheic keratosis growth. You may experience some mild discomfort or a stinging sensation during the freezing process, but this typically subsides quickly.

Post-treatment care is crucial for optimizing healing and minimizing potential complications. Your dermatologist will provide you with specific instructions on how to care for the treated area, including keeping it clean, avoiding picking or scratching, and applying any suggested ointments or dressings.

By seeking professional advice, you can make an informed decision that prioritizes your skin health and overall well-being.

Its precision, effectiveness, and minimal downtime make it an attractive choice in the quest for clear, healthy skin.

- Laser therapy

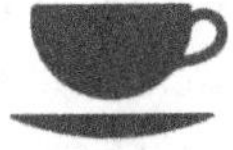

This procedure aids in the reduction or elimination of seborrheic keratosis lesions, which are benign growths that often appear as rough, scaly patches on the skin.

The targeted nature of laser beams allows for the selective removal of afflicted tissue without causing damage to the surrounding healthy skin. This attribute proves particularly beneficial for mature women, as it minimizes the risk of scarring and ensures a more seamless healing process.

By precisely targeting seborrheic keratosis lesions, lasers can effectively reduce or eliminate the discolored, raised, or rough patches characterizing this condition. This ultimately translates into a smoother, more even complexion that enhances the overall appearance of the skin.

We must also acknowledge the unique needs of mature women when considering treatment options for seborrheic keratosis. As we age, our skin becomes more delicate and susceptible to damage. Traditional methods, such as scraping or freezing off the lesions, can, at times, be too harsh for mature skin, potentially leading to inflammation, scarring, or prolonged recovery times.

Collagen, a vital protein responsible for skin elasticity, tends to diminish as we age, resulting in sagging or drooping skin. By utilizing laser treatment for seborrheic keratosis, mature women can not only target the condition but simultaneously promote the rejuvenation of their skin, leading to a more youthful and radiant appearance.

However, it should only be administered by a qualified dermatologist who possesses the necessary expertise and experience in utilizing lasers for dermatological conditions. Proper pre-treatment consultation, including a comprehensive skin evaluation, will ensure that the treatment plan is tailored to suit individual needs, minimizing any potential risks or complications.

Its precision, superior cosmetic outcomes, gentle approach, and collagen-stimulating properties make it an ideal choice for this specific demographic.

- Surgical removal

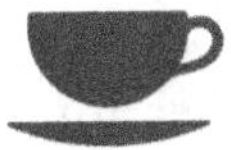

Seborrheic keratosis is a common skin condition that manifests as growths on the skin. These growths are typically brown or black in color and have a waxy or scaly texture. While they are generally harmless, seborrheic keratoses can be unattractive and cause considerable distress to mature women.

It involves the physical removal of the growths through various techniques, which I will further discuss in this essay.

This procedure involves scraping off the growth with a curette, a small, sharp instrument, and then using electrocautery or a high-frequency electrical current to seal the wound. The advantage of this technique is that it can be performed in an outpatient setting, and it is generally well-tolerated by patients. However, there is a possibility of scarring, so it is crucial that you have realistic expectations and discuss this with your dermatologist prior to the procedure.

As the name suggests, this procedure involves the shaving off of the growth using a scalpel. Unlike curettage and desiccation, shave excision does not involve sealing the wound with electrocautery. Following the excision, the wound is left to heal on its own. This technique is effective in removing smaller or superficial growths and is relatively quick to perform. However, as with any surgical procedure, there is a risk of infection or scarring, and meticulous wound care post-procedure is essential.

Liquid nitrogen is applied to the growth, causing it to freeze and subsequently fall off. Cryosurgery is relatively fast, and it can be used to treat multiple growths in one session. However, this technique may cause temporary discoloration and swelling around the treated area, and there is a probability of residual skin changes or scarring. Therefore, it is crucial to discuss the potential risks and benefits with your dermatologist.

Laser treatment involves using high-intensity light beams to destroy and vaporize the growth. This technique offers precision and minimal scarring compared to other surgical methods. However, laser therapy may not be suitable for all types of seborrheic keratosis, and it may require multiple sessions to achieve satisfactory results.

Curettage and desiccation, shave excision, cryosurgery, and laser therapy are among the surgical approaches available. As a professional dermatologist, it is essential to assess the suitability of each method based on the characteristics and severity of your condition. Remember to consult with a dermatologist to determine the most appropriate treatment option for your specific case and to discuss possible risks and benefits. With the right treatment, you can achieve clear, rejuvenated skin and restore your confidence.

- Home remedies and natural treatments

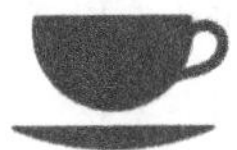

Seborrheic keratosis is a common skin condition that primarily affects mature women. Characterized by the appearance of raised, wart-like growths on different areas of the body, seborrheic keratosis can be aesthetically distressing. By exploring various natural remedies, this guide will provide mature women with options to help improve the appearance and health of their skin.

Aloe Vera:

One natural remedy that has gained popularity for treating seborrheic keratosis is Aloe vera. Known for its soothing and healing properties, Aloe vera can be applied topically to affected areas. The gel extracted from the Aloe vera plant contains several bioactive compounds, such as vitamins, minerals, glycoproteins, and polysaccharides, all of which have been recognized for their regenerative and anti-inflammatory effects on the skin. Regular application of Aloe vera gel can result in a reduction in the size and coloration of seborrheic keratosis, promoting clearer and healthier-looking skin.

Apple Cider Vinegar:

Apple cider vinegar is another popular natural remedy for seborrheic keratosis. Its acidic properties make it an effective treatment option for skin conditions. When applied directly to affected areas, the acetic acid present in apple cider vinegar helps break down the excessive keratin that accumulates in seborrheic keratosis growths, ultimately leading to their gradual disappearance. However, it is important to dilute apple cider vinegar before application to prevent skin irritations or burns. Patients should also exercise caution if applying apple cider vinegar to areas around the eyes or on sensitive skin.

Tea Tree Oil:

Tea tree oil has been used for centuries in traditional medicine for its antifungal, antibacterial, and anti-inflammatory properties. When it comes to seborrheic keratosis, tea tree oil can help reduce inflammation, itching, and redness associated with the condition. Diluting tea tree oil and applying it topically to affected areas can assist in flattening seborrheic keratosis growths and lightening their appearance. It is important to note that a patch test should be conducted on a small area of skin before applying tea tree oil directly to larger affected areas to avoid any potential adverse reactions.

Coconut Oil:

An increasingly popular remedy for various skin conditions, including seborrheic keratosis, is coconut oil. Coconut oil is known for its moisturizing and nourishing properties, which can help soften the skin and potentially reduce the appearance of the growths. Daily application of virgin coconut oil can aid in improving the overall texture and coloration of the skin, making the seborrheic keratosis lesions less prominent. Additionally, coconut oil contains antioxidants that may help protect against inflammation and oxidative stress caused by the condition.

Seborrheic keratosis can be challenging for mature women, as it often impacts their self-confidence and overall appearance. Aloe vera, apple cider vinegar, tea tree oil, and coconut oil are just a few of the many natural options available for managing seborrheic keratosis. It is important to remember that results may vary, and consulting with a dermatologist is recommended before trying any new treatment approach. By exploring these natural remedies, mature women can take control of their skin health and enjoy a clearer and more youthful complexion.

Chapter 5: Prevention and Management

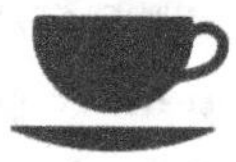

- Sun protection strategies

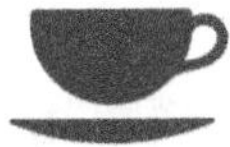

In the pursuit of clear and healthy skin, sun protection stands as a fundamental pillar for women of all ages. However, for mature women, it becomes even more crucial, given the increased vulnerability to various dermatological conditions.

Ultraviolet Radiation: The Culprit:

Before diving into preventive measures, it is essential to understand the underlying cause of Seborrheic Keratosis. This harmless, non-cancerous skin growth often manifests as slightly raised, thick, and waxy areas with a color ranging from light tan to dark brown. Chronic exposure to ultraviolet (UV) radiation, particularly UVB and UVA rays, plays a significant role in the development and worsening of these lesions.

Physical Sunscreen as an Imperative:

Utilizing sunscreens with adequate sun protection factor (SPF) is an essential aspect of any sun protection strategy. Physical sunscreens, which contain active mineral ingredients like titanium dioxide or zinc oxide, act as a physical barrier, reflecting and scattering UV radiation away from the skin. They are particularly advantageous for mature women with Seborrheic Keratosis, as they provide broad-spectrum protection against both UVA and UVB rays. Moreover, physical sunscreens are typically less irritating and less likely to cause adverse reactions in individuals with sensitive skin.

Proper Application for Optimal Protection:

Merely owning sunscreen is not enough; proper application is equally important. When using physical sunscreen, a sufficient amount should be applied evenly to all sun-exposed areas, including the face, neck, décolletage, and hands. It is advisable to apply sunscreen at least 15 minutes before sun exposure to allow it to bind to the skin and start providing protection. Reapplication every two hours, or immediately after swimming or vigorous sweating, will maximize the effectiveness of the sunscreen in preventing the worsening of Seborrheic Keratosis lesions.

Additional Protective Measures:

In addition to sunscreen, mature women should embrace other protective measures to prevent and manage Seborrheic Keratosis. Wearing protective clothing, such as broad-brimmed hats, long-sleeved shirts, and pants with a tightly woven fabric, offers a physical barrier against harmful UV radiation. Those who engage in outdoor activities for an extended period should consider seeking shade, especially during peak sunlight hours. Finally, sunglasses with UV protection should be worn to safeguard the delicate skin around the eyes.

Cumulative Sun Exposure versus Essential Sun Exposure:

While it is crucial to protect the skin from excessive sun exposure, it is equally important not to restrict oneself entirely from the benefits of essential sun exposure. Balanced exposure to sunlight, particularly in the morning or late afternoon, helps the body synthesize vitamin D, which is essential for overall health. Consulting with a dermatologist or healthcare provider can provide guidance on the appropriate amount of sun exposure required, given an individual's specific circumstances.

This entails utilizing physical sunscreens with adequate SPF, applying them generously and regularly, and complementing them with protective clothing, seeking shade, and wearing sunglasses. Balancing essential sun exposure with the need for photo-protection contributes to maintaining clear and healthy skin throughout the aging process. By adhering to these guidelines, mature women can actively take charge of their skin health and enjoy the benefits of a radiant complexion for years to come.

- Skincare routines for mature women

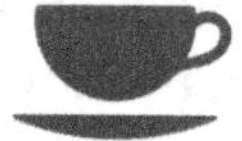

Through a comprehensive skincare routine, mature women can effectively address and manage this condition, ensuring healthy and radiant skin.

Seborrheic keratosis is a benign skin growth that often presents as raised, wart-like lesions. While this condition is generally harmless, it can still cause significant distress and affect one's self-esteem due to its highly visible nature. Therefore, adopting a skincare routine that aims at both prevention and management of seborrheic keratosis becomes crucial for mature women.

1. Cleansing: The first step in any skincare routine is proper cleansing. Mature women should opt for a gentle, non-abrasive cleanser that is specifically formulated for their skin type. Cleansing the face twice daily using lukewarm water and a targeted cleanser helps remove impurities, excess oil, and dead skin cells, all factors that can contribute to the development of skin conditions such as seborrheic keratosis.

2. Exfoliation: Exfoliating the skin is essential to promote the turnover of new skin cells and prevent the accumulation of dead skin cells, which can enhance the appearance of seborrheic keratosis. However, it is crucial to choose gentle exfoliators that do not irritate or damage the skin. Chemical exfoliants containing ingredients like salicylic acid or alpha-hydroxy acids can be beneficial in managing the condition effectively.

3. Moisturization: As the skin ages, it tends to become drier and may lose its natural ability to retain moisture. Therefore, incorporating a hydrating moisturizer into the skincare routine is essential to maintain the skin's suppleness and prevent the occurrence of seborrheic keratosis. Look for moisturizers with ingredients such as hyaluronic acid, ceramides, or glycerin, which help restore the skin's moisture barrier.

4. Sun protection: Sun exposure can exacerbate the development and appearance of seborrheic keratosis. Therefore, mature women should prioritize sun protection as an essential component of their skincare routine. The regular use of broad-spectrum sunscreen with a high Sun Protection Factor (SPF) of 30 or above, along with protective clothing and accessories, can help shield the skin from harmful UV rays and minimize the risk of developing seborrheic keratosis.

5. Nourishing the skin: Incorporating serums and treatments into the skincare routine can provide additional benefits in preventing and managing seborrheic keratosis. Look for products that contain antioxidants, such as vitamin C or E, which can neutralize free radicals and protect the skin. Additionally, the use of retinoids or retinol-based products can aid in promoting cell turnover and maintaining a youthful appearance.

It is important to highlight that skincare routines should go beyond external care and include the adoption of a healthy lifestyle. Adequate hydration, regular exercise, a balanced diet, and stress management are all vital contributors to maintaining healthy skin. These holistic approaches help support the skin's overall health, resilience, and ability to repair itself, aiding in the prevention and management of conditions like seborrheic keratosis.

Through a proper cleansing and exfoliation routine, adequate moisturization, sun protection, and the use of nourishing serums, mature women can enhance their skin's health, reduce the occurrence of seborrheic keratosis, and promote a radiant and clear complexion. Additionally, adopting a healthy lifestyle and self-care practices further contribute to maintaining healthy and youthful-looking skin.

- Monitoring and self-examination

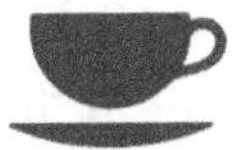

By regularly monitoring their skin and performing self-examinations, women can identify any changes in their skin and seek appropriate medical attention promptly.

As a dermatologist, I cannot stress enough the importance of monitoring one's skin. By closely observing any changes that may occur, individuals can catch potential issues early on, allowing for earlier treatment and better overall prognosis. This is particularly crucial for mature women since they may be at a higher risk of developing Seborrheic keratosis due to hormonal changes and cumulative sun exposure over the years.

Seborrheic keratosis is a common skin condition characterized by benign growths on the skin's surface. These growths often appear as rough, scaly patches that range in color from white or yellow to brown or black.

When performing self-examinations for Seborrheic keratosis, it is important to be thorough and systematic. Start by undressing and standing in front of a mirror in a well-lit room. Examine your skin from head to toe, paying close attention to areas where Seborrheic keratosis commonly occur, such as the face, neck, chest, back, and extremities. Use a handheld mirror to inspect hard-to-see areas like the back of your neck or between your toes.

While conducting self-examinations, be on the lookout for any changes in the color, size, shape, or texture of existing Seborrheic keratosis lesions. Additionally, take note of any new growths that may have appeared. If you notice any drastic changes or are unsure about a particular lesion, it is crucial to consult a dermatologist for further evaluation. They can assess the lesion and determine if any additional tests or treatments are necessary.

In addition to self-examinations, regular monitoring of the skin is paramount. By being attentive to your skin's appearance and any changes that may occur, you can effectively track the progress of Seborrheic keratosis and address any concerns promptly. Having a good understanding of your own skin is crucial for early detection and management of this condition.

To further aid in self-examinations and monitoring, it is helpful to maintain a record of any changes observed. This can be achieved through taking photographs of suspicious lesions or using a body map to indicate the location and characteristics of specific growths. By having documentation, it becomes easier to track any changes over time and discuss them with a dermatologist, if necessary.

Lastly, it is important to emphasize that self-examinations and monitoring should not replace regular visits to a dermatologist. While self-examinations empower individuals to be proactive about their skin health, dermatologists have the expertise necessary to diagnose and effectively manage Seborrheic keratosis.

By being vigilant about any changes in their skin and regularly performing self-examinations, women can detect potential issues early on and seek appropriate medical attention. Remember to be thorough, systematic, and seek professional guidance when needed.

- Follow-up care after treatment

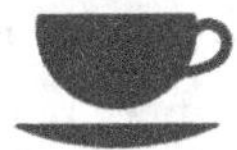

Seborrheic keratosis is a common skin condition that affects many mature women. While treatment options for seborrheic keratosis are effective in managing the condition, it is important to keep in mind that follow-up care is crucial to maintain clear and healthy skin.

Even after successful treatment, it is essential to keep a close eye on the skin and observe if any new lesions appear. Regular self-examinations can help identify any changes or abnormalities, and immediate medical attention should be sought if any concerning signs are observed. By closely monitoring the skin, dermatologists can intervene early if the condition shows signs of recurrence or if any suspicious features indicate a different underlying condition.

Furthermore, after treatment for seborrheic keratosis, it is important to maintain a comprehensive skincare routine. This includes regular cleansing, moisturizing, and sun protection to keep the skin healthy and minimize the chances of developing new lesions or complications. Using gentle cleansers that do not irritate the skin is crucial, as seborrheic keratosis-prone skin can be sensitive. Additionally, applying moisturizers can improve the overall texture and appearance of the skin.

Sun protection is especially vital in follow-up care for seborrheic keratosis. Mature women should be advised to use broad-spectrum sunscreen with a high sun protection factor (SPF) on a daily basis, regardless of the weather conditions.

Exposure to the sun's harmful ultraviolet (UV) rays can exacerbate the condition and increase the risk of further development of seborrheic keratosis. Wearing appropriate clothing, such as wide-brimmed hats and protective clothing, can also provide an extra layer of defense against UV rays.

Apart from skincare routines, regular check-ups with a dermatologist are essential for follow-up care. These visits allow the professional to assess the response to treatment and ensure optimal management of seborrheic keratosis. During these appointments, the dermatologist can carefully examine the skin, address any concerns, and propose additional treatment options if required. Moreover, regular follow-up appointments contribute to building a strong patient-doctor relationship, which is important for effective long-term management of seborrheic keratosis.

In terms of psychological well-being, follow-up care should also include discussions about the emotional impact of seborrheic keratosis. Skin conditions can affect one's self-esteem and body image, especially among mature women who may already be grappling with other age-related changes. Providing emotional support, educating patients about the benign nature of seborrheic keratosis, and informing them about various cosmetic procedures to address associated concerns can go a long way in enhancing overall patient satisfaction and well-being.

By closely monitoring skin changes, adhering to a comprehensive skincare routine, utilizing sun protection measures, and attending regular dermatologist visits, patients can optimize their long-term management of seborrheic keratosis. Additionally, addressing emotional concerns and providing necessary support can contribute to a positive patient experience. With proper follow-up care, mature women can enjoy clear and radiant skin, enhancing their overall quality of life.

Conclusion

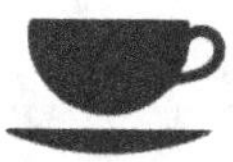

- Recap of key points about seborrheic keratosis in mature women

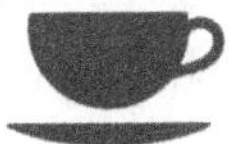

Seborrheic keratosis is a common skin condition that affects mature women. Throughout this book, we have explored various aspects of seborrheic keratosis and discussed its causes, symptoms, and treatment options. In this section, we will recap the key points related to seborrheic keratosis in mature women.

First and foremost, it is important to understand that seborrheic keratosis is a noncancerous growth that appears on the skin. The exact cause of this condition is still unknown, but it is believed to be linked to genetic factors and changes in hormone levels that occur during the aging process.

One key characteristic of seborrheic keratosis is the presence of raised, waxy, and scaly growths on the skin. These growths are usually brown, black, or tan in color and can vary in size and shape. They are most commonly found on areas of the body that are exposed to the sun, such as the face, chest, and back.

Although seborrheic keratosis is a benign condition, it can cause cosmetic concerns for many mature women. These growths can be unsightly and may affect one's self-esteem. Therefore, it is important to be aware of the available treatment options.

One effective treatment for seborrheic keratosis is cryotherapy, which involves freezing the growths with liquid nitrogen. This causes the growths to fall off, allowing new skin to regenerate. Cryotherapy is a quick and relatively painless procedure that can be performed in a dermatologist's office.

Another treatment option is curettage, which involves scraping off the growths using a special instrument called a curette. This procedure can be combined with cryotherapy to ensure complete removal of the growth.

In addition to these treatment options, there are also home remedies and topical treatments available for managing seborrheic keratosis. These include the use of apple cider vinegar, hydrogen peroxide, and over-the-counter creams or lotions containing ingredients such as salicylic acid or alpha-hydroxy acids. However, it is important to consult with a dermatologist before trying any home remedies to ensure their safety and effectiveness.

It is worth noting that seborrheic keratosis is a benign condition and does not pose any serious health risks. However, it is recommended to have any new growths or changes in existing growths evaluated by a dermatologist to rule out any other skin conditions that may require further medical attention.

It is characterized by raised, waxy growths on the skin and is believed to be linked to genetic and hormonal factors. Treatment options for seborrheic keratosis include cryotherapy, curettage, home remedies, and topical treatments. Remember to consult with a dermatologist for a proper diagnosis and personalized treatment plan. By understanding and addressing this condition, mature women can achieve clear and healthy skin.

- Importance of early detection and treatment

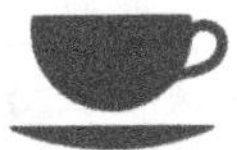

This common skin condition can have a noticeable impact on an individual's physical appearance and emotional well-being. In this final chapter, we have explored various aspects related to seborrheic keratosis, including its causes, prevalence in mature women, and potential treatment options.

The path to clear skin at any age is paved with early detection. By identifying seborrheic keratosis at its earliest stages, mature women can ensure timely intervention and reduce the severity of the condition. Early detection allows dermatologists to develop personalized treatment plans that address the specific needs of each patient. This is crucial as seborrheic keratosis can vary in its presentation and severity.

Furthermore, addressing seborrheic keratosis promptly can also aid in preventing potential complications. Although this skin condition is typically harmless, it can sometimes resemble other, more serious skin conditions. Early detection enables dermatologists to differentiate between seborrheic keratosis and potentially malignant skin growths such as melanoma. This differentiation is vital for accurate diagnosis and appropriate treatment.

Treatment also plays a pivotal role in managing seborrheic keratosis in mature women. The treatment options can vary depending on the nature and extent of the keratoses. It is essential for dermatologists to assess each patient's unique situation and provide tailored treatment recommendations. Early treatment not only helps individuals maintain clear skin but also prevents further recurrence and potential complications.

One of the most common treatment options for seborrheic keratosis is cryotherapy. This technique involves freezing the keratosis using liquid nitrogen, effectively destroying the unwanted growths. Cryotherapy is a quick and relatively painless procedure, making it an attractive option for mature women seeking to remove their keratoses.

Another treatment modality that may be used for seborrheic keratosis is curettage. Dermatologists employ a sharp instrument called a curette to scrape off the affected area gently. This method ensures complete removal of the keratosis and allows for subsequent healing. Curettage is often combined with electrodessication, which involves using an electric current to stop bleeding and promote skin healing.

Furthermore, topical creams containing ingredients such as salicylic acid or glycolic acid may also be recommended. These creams help soften the keratoses, improve their appearance, and promote exfoliation over time. Although this treatment option may take longer to yield visible results compared to cryotherapy or curettage, it offers a non-invasive alternative for mature women seeking less aggressive interventions.

Early intervention allows dermatologists to develop personalized treatment plans, accurately differentiate between seborrheic keratosis and potentially malignant skin growths, and prevent potential complications. Treatment options such as cryotherapy, curettage, and topical creams provide various alternatives for removing the keratoses and maintaining overall skin health. By placing importance on early detection and timely treatment, mature women can confidently embrace their age while retaining radiant and healthy-looking skin.

61

- Encouragement for ongoing skin health habits and regular check-ups.

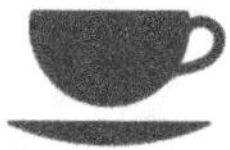

As a professional dermatologist, I understand the importance of ongoing skin health habits and regular check-ups for maintaining clear and radiant skin, especially for mature women who may be more prone to certain skin conditions, such as seborrheic keratosis. In this essay, I will offer encouragement and advice to help mature women develop consistent skin care habits, as well as stress the significance of regular check-ups with a dermatologist.

Taking care of your skin should be a lifelong commitment, and it becomes increasingly important as we age. Mature skin often experiences changes in texture, tone, and elasticity. It may also become more susceptible to developing various skin conditions. By establishing good skin care habits, you can help prevent or minimize such issues and maintain skin that not only looks healthy but also feels smooth and supple.

First and foremost, a proper daily skin care routine is essential to ongoing skin health. This routine should include cleansing, moisturizing, and protecting the skin from harmful ultraviolet (UV) radiation. Cleansing the skin twice daily, using a gentle cleanser suitable for your skin type, helps remove dirt, oil, and environmental pollutants. This step helps to unclog pores and prevent blemishes.

Moisturizing is particularly important for mature women, as aging skin tends to be drier and more prone to dehydration.

Choose a moisturizer that suits your skin type and is designed specifically for mature skin. Look for key ingredients such as hyaluronic acid, ceramides, and antioxidants, which help to hydrate, repair, and protect the skin.

Protecting your skin from UV radiation is crucial in order to prevent premature aging, skin damage, and even the development of skin cancer. Apply a broad-spectrum sunscreen with a minimum SPF of 30 daily, even on cloudy days, and reapply every two hours when exposed to direct sunlight.

In addition to a daily skin care routine, it is important to invest in specialized treatments that target the specific concerns of mature skin. Consider incorporating products that contain retinol, peptides, or growth factors, as they can help reduce the appearance of fine lines, wrinkles, and age spots. Additionally, incorporating a regular exfoliation routine can help to remove dead skin cells and stimulate cell turnover, promoting a vibrant and youthful complexion.

While developing and maintaining a proper skin care routine is essential, regular check-ups with a dermatologist play an equally important role in ongoing skin health for mature women. Dermatologists are trained to identify and diagnose various skin conditions, often before they become visible or develop into something serious. Regular check-ups allow dermatologists to assess any changes in your skin and provide appropriate treatment or preventive measures.

During a dermatologist visit, a professional will not only perform a thorough examination of your skin but also give personalized recommendations for your concerns. These recommendations may include prescription medications, topical treatments, in-office procedures, or lifestyle modifications.

Furthermore, dermatologists have access to advanced diagnostic tools and treatments that can effectively address specific skin concerns, such as seborrheic keratosis. These benign skin growths often occur in mature individuals and can appear as rough, scaly patches that can be mistaken for other more serious skin conditions. Dermatologists can not only provide accurate diagnoses but also offer the most appropriate treatment options, which may include cryotherapy, electrosurgery, or prescription creams.

Establishing a consistent daily skin care routine, including cleansing, moisturizing, and sun protection, is key. Additionally, incorporating specialized treatments and seeking the guidance of a dermatologist further supports ongoing skin health. By committing to these practices, mature women can enjoy healthy, glowing skin well into their later years. Keep in mind that prevention, early detection, and professional advice are always the best approaches to achieving and maintaining vibrant and youthful skin.